GAST

AND DIABETES

COOKBOOK

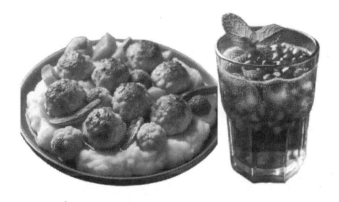

Quick and Easy Delicious Meals to

Manage Gastroparesis and Diabetes

Symptoms

Noreen Hart

Copyright © 2024 by Noreen Hart

TABLE OF CONTENT

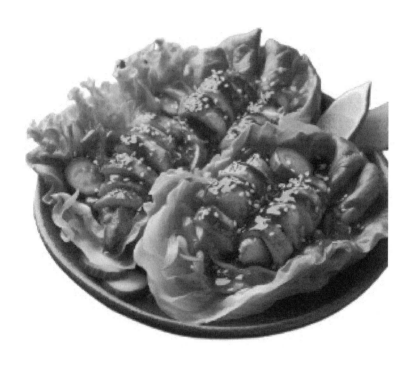

Disclaimer

The information provided in this cookbook is for educational and informational purposes only. It is not intended to be a substitute for professional medical advice, diagnosis, or treatment.

Always seek the advice of your physician or other qualified health provider with any questions you may have regarding a medical condition.

The recipes and dietary suggestions included are based on general principles and may not be suitable for everyone.

Individual dietary needs and health conditions vary, and it is essential to consult with a healthcare professional before making significant changes to your diet.

The author and publisher disclaim responsibility for any effects resulting directly or indirectly from the use or misuse of the information provided in this cookbook.

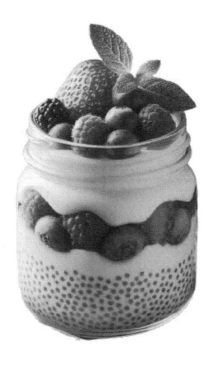

Introduction

Have you ever felt like your body was betraying you, making it difficult to enjoy the simple pleasures of a delicious meal?

Does the thought of planning and preparing nourishing dishes leave you feeling overwhelmed and discouraged?

You are not alone! Gastroparesis, a condition marked by delayed gastric emptying, and diabetes, a metabolic disorder affecting blood sugar regulation, can turn mealtimes into a source of discomfort and frustration.

But fear not, for this book is your guide to reclaiming the pleasure of eating while navigating these challenges with grace and resilience. It is a roadmap to empowering yourself and taking control of your well-being.

Within these pages, you'll discover a harmonious blend of strategies and recipes tailored specifically for those facing the unique intersection of these two conditions.

Unlike generic solutions you've probably come across so far, this book is meticulously designed with your specific needs in mind. You'll learn the principles of the gastroparesis diet and the benefits it can bring, while also exploring the dietary considerations for managing diabetes. Each recipe is a carefully crafted masterpiece of flavor, nutrition, and digestibility, ensuring that every bite nourishes both your body and your soul.

Imagine a world where every bite is a celebration of flavor and nourishment, where you can savor the culinary delights without the unwanted side effects.

This book is a harmonious blend of deliciousness and health. It is your key to unlocking that reality, offering a comprehensive approach to managing gastroparesis and diabetes through thoughtfully crafted recipes and practical strategies.

From start to finish, you'll be guided through the principles of the gastroparesis diet, equipping you with the knowledge and tools to make informed choices that promote your overall health and quality of life.

But this book is more than just a practical guide; it's a reminder that you are not alone in this journey, we're in it together, every step of the way.

Together, we'll embark on a culinary adventure that celebrates the joys of good food while managing the challenges of gastroparesis and diabetes with grace and resilience.

So, let's begin this transformative journey, where every bite is a step towards a healthier, more vibrant you.

In the pages ahead, you'll discover the principles of the gastroparesis and diabetes diet, the benefits it can bring, and a collection of delectable recipes that will tantalize your taste buds while nourishing your body and soul.

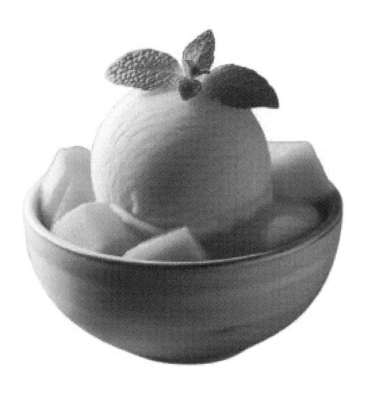

CHAPTER 1

Principles of the Diabetic Gastroparesis Diet

1. **Low-Fiber Foods:** Opt for easily digestible foods low in fiber to reduce strain on your digestive system. This includes refined grains, well-cooked vegetables without skins or seeds, and tender lean meats.

2. **Small, Frequent Meals:** Rather than large meals, aim for smaller, more frequent meals throughout the day. This helps prevent overloading your stomach, leading to better digestion and less discomfort.

3. **Soft and Moist Foods:** Choose foods that are soft, moist, and easy to chew and swallow. This can include pureed foods, smoothies, soups, and stews that are gentle on your stomach.

4. **Limited Fat Content:** Reduce the amount of fat in your diet, especially saturated and trans fats, as they can slow down digestion and exacerbate gastroparesis symptoms.

Opt for lean protein sources and healthier fats like those found in avocados and nuts.

5. **Avoiding Trigger Foods:** Identify and avoid foods that trigger symptoms such as nausea, bloating, and discomfort.

   Common triggers include spicy foods, carbonated beverages, caffeine, and high-fat or greasy foods.

6. **Hydration:** Stay well-hydrated by drinking plenty of fluids, preferably water or herbal teas. Avoid sugary drinks and alcohol, which can aggravate gastroparesis symptoms.

7. **Balanced Nutrition:** Despite dietary restrictions, strive for a balanced diet that includes essential nutrients like vitamins, minerals, and protein.

   Incorporate nutrient-dense foods such as fruits, vegetables, lean proteins, and whole grains when possible.

These principles form the foundation of a gastroparesis-friendly diet, offering practical strategies to manage symptoms and promote overall health.

By following these guidelines and making mindful food choices, you can support your well-being and enhance your quality of life.

Benefits of Diabetic Gastroparesis Diet

1. **Symptom Management:** One of the primary benefits of the Gastroparesis and Diabetes Diet is effective symptom management. By selecting foods gentle on the digestive system and avoiding triggers, you can alleviate symptoms such as nausea, bloating, abdominal pain, and reflux, while also stabilizing blood sugar levels.

2. **Improved Digestion:** The diet emphasizes easily digestible foods, reducing digestive discomfort and promoting smoother digestion. This can lead to fewer episodes of stomach fullness, early satiety, delayed gastric emptying, and fluctuations in blood sugar levels.

3. **Stable Blood Sugar Levels:** For individuals managing both gastroparesis and diabetes, following a Gastroparesis and Diabetes Diet helps stabilize blood sugar levels. Through smaller, frequent meals and low-glycemic index foods, you

can better manage glucose levels and prevent spikes and crashes, while also supporting digestive health.

4. **Enhanced Nutrient Absorption:** The diet focuses on nutrient-dense foods rich in vitamins, minerals, and essential nutrients. This supports optimal nutrient absorption, ensuring your body receives vital elements necessary for overall health, while also considering diabetic dietary restrictions.

5. **Weight Management:** Promoting portion control and mindful eating, the Gastroparesis and Diabetes Diet aids in weight management. It prevents overeating while providing adequate nutrition, facilitating easier maintenance of a healthy weight, and supporting blood sugar control.

6. **Increased Energy Levels:** Promoting portion control and mindful eating, the Gastroparesis and Diabetes Diet aids in weight management. It prevents overeating while providing adequate nutrition, facilitating easier maintenance of a healthy weight, and supporting blood sugar control.

7. **Improved Quality of Life:** Ultimately, following a Gastroparesis and Diabetes Diet leads to an

improved quality of life. By managing symptoms effectively, supporting digestion, stabilizing blood sugar, and promoting overall health, individuals can enjoy a higher level of well-being and comfort in their daily lives, despite the challenges of both conditions.

Foods to Eat

Lean Proteins: Base your meals around lean protein sources such as skinless poultry, fish, tofu, and legumes. These proteins are easier to digest and provide essential amino acids for muscle health, while also helping to manage blood sugar levels.

Soft Cooked Vegetables: Opt for soft cooked vegetables like carrots, squash, green beans, and spinach. Steaming or simmering these vegetables until tender makes them easier to digest while retaining their nutritional value, making them suitable for individuals with both conditions.

Fruits: Choose soft and easy-to-chew fruits such as melons, peaches, and applesauce. Avoid fruits with tough skins or seeds that may be difficult to digest, while also considering their impact on blood sugar levels.

Low-Fiber Grains: Incorporate low-fiber grains like white rice, refined pasta, oatmeal, and couscous into your meals. These grains are gentler on the stomach and promote better digestion, while also being mindful of their glycemic index for diabetes management.

Healthy Fats: Include healthy fats from sources like avocados, olive oil, nuts, and seeds to support overall health. These fats provide essential nutrients and energy without burdening the digestive system or negatively impacting blood sugar levels.

Dairy Alternatives: For those with lactose intolerance or a preference for dairy alternatives, choose lactose-free milk, yogurt, and cheese. Plant-based options like almond milk and coconut yogurt are excellent choices suitable for both conditions.

Smooth Nut Butters: Enjoy smooth nut butters made from almonds, peanuts, or cashews. Spread them on toast, crackers, or incorporate them into smoothies for a nutritious boost, while being mindful of portion sizes and carbohydrate content for diabetes control.

Soups and Broths: Warm, soothing soups and broths made from clear liquids, vegetables, and lean proteins are ideal for easy digestion and hydration, making them suitable for individuals managing both gastroparesis and diabetes.

Foods to Avoid

High-Fiber Foods: Steer clear of high-fiber foods like whole grains, raw vegetables, and fruits with skins or seeds. These options can be difficult to digest and may cause discomfort, while also impacting blood sugar levels.

Tough Meats: Avoid tough cuts of meat and processed meats that are hard to chew and digest. Instead, opt for tender cuts or lean proteins that are easier on your stomach, and consider their impact on blood sugar management.

Greasy or Fried Foods: Limit greasy or fried foods as they can slow down digestion and lead to bloating and discomfort. Choose baked, grilled, or steamed options instead, while also considering their effect on blood lipid levels and diabetes control.

Spicy Foods: Skip spicy foods that can irritate the digestive tract and trigger symptoms like heartburn and acid reflux. Opt for milder seasonings and herbs to flavor your meals, considering their potential impact on blood sugar and digestive health.

High-Fat Foods: Cut back on high-fat foods such as creamy sauces, butter, and rich desserts. These can contribute to digestive sluggishness and may worsen gastroparesis symptoms, while also affecting blood lipid levels and insulin sensitivity in diabetes management.

Carbonated Beverages: Avoid carbonated beverages such as sparkling water and soda; they can cause gas and bloating. Stick to still water, herbal teas, and non-carbonated drinks to stay hydrated without impacting blood sugar levels or aggravating digestive issues.

Alcohol and Caffeine: Limit alcohol consumption as it can irritate the stomach lining and disrupt digestion. Likewise, reduce intake of caffeinated beverages like coffee and tea, which can stimulate gastric acid production and affect blood sugar levels and insulin sensitivity.

Large Meals: Steer clear of large meals that can overwhelm your digestive system. Break down your daily intake into smaller, more frequent meals for better digestion, while also considering their impact on blood sugar control and insulin management.

Comprehensive Shopping List for Diabetic Gastroparesis Diet

Proteins:

- Skinless chicken breasts
- Turkey breast slices
- Fish filets (e.g., cod, salmon)
- Tofu or tempeh
- Canned tuna or salmon (in water)
- Lentils or chickpeas (canned or dried)
- Lean cuts of beef or pork (tender and easy to digest)
- Eggs or egg whites

Soft Cooked Vegetables:

- Carrots
- Zucchini
- Spinach (fresh or frozen)
- Green beans

- Peas (canned or frozen)
- Canned pumpkin or squash
- Bell peppers
- Cucumbers
- Tomatoes

Fruits:

- Applesauce (unsweetened)
- Melons (e.g., cantaloupe, honeydew)
- Peaches (canned in juice)
- Avocado
- Pears (canned in water)
- Berries (strawberries, blueberries, raspberries)

Low-Fiber Grains:

- White rice (instant or regular)
- Refined pasta (e.g., spaghetti, penne)
- Oatmeal (quick-cooking or rolled oats)
- Couscous
- White bread or rolls (low-fiber)
- Quinoa
- Barley
- Bulgur

Healthy Fats:

- Avocado
- Olive oil
- Almond butter or peanut butter (smooth)
- Nuts (e.g., almonds, walnuts)
- Seeds (e.g., chia seeds, sunflower seeds)
- Fatty fish (mackerel, sardines)

Dairy Alternatives:

- Lactose-free milk (cow's milk or plant-based)
- Yogurt (low-fat, plain, or lactose-free)
- Cheese (low-fat varieties)
- Plant-based milk (e.g., coconut milk/almond milk,)
- Unsweetened soy or coconut yogurt

Soups and Broths:

- Low-sodium chicken or vegetable broth
- Canned soups (low-fat, low-sodium)
- Broth-based soups (e.g., chicken noodle, tomato)

Herbs and Spices:

- Salt (in moderation)

- Pepper
- Basil
- Oregano
- Ginger (fresh or ground)
- Cinnamon
- Turmeric
- Garlic
- Cilantro

Beverages:

- Water
- Herbal teas (e.g., chamomile, peppermint)
- Green tea
- Unsweetened fruit juices (diluted if needed)
- Sports drinks (electrolyte-replenishing, low-sugar)

Snacks and Treats:

- Smoothies (made with low-fiber fruits and yogurt)
- Gelatin desserts (sugar-free)
- Applesauce cups (individual servings)
- Low-fat crackers or pretzels
- Sugar-free dark chocolate

CHAPTER 2

Breakfast Recipes for Gastroparesis Diet

Vanilla Chia Pudding

- **Preparation Time:** 5 minutes (plus 4 hours chilling time)
- **Serves:** 2

Ingredients:

- 1/4 cup chia seeds
- 1 cup unsweetened almond milk or coconut milk
- 1/2 teaspoon vanilla extract
- 1/4 teaspoon ground cinnamon (optional)

Nutritional Information: Calories: 185, Carbs: 14g, Fiber: 10g, Protein: 5g, Fat: 11g

Instructions:

1. In a jar or bowl, combine the chia seeds, unsweetened non-dairy milk, vanilla extract, and cinnamon (if using).

2. Stir well to combine and break up any clumps of chia seeds.

3. Cover and refrigerate for at least 4 hours, or overnight, stirring occasionally to prevent the chia from clumping.

4. Once thickened to a pudding-like consistency, give it a final stir before serving.

Serving Suggestions:

- Top with fresh berries, sliced almonds, or a dollop of unsweetened yogurt for added flavor and nutrition. You can also serve it alongside jicama "toast" or cucumber slices for a low-carb accompaniment.

Warm Rice Cereal with Cinnamon

- **Preparation Time:** 15 minutes
- **Serves:** 2

Ingredients:

- 1/2 cup white rice
- 1 cup water

- 1 cup almond milk
- 1/2 teaspoon ground cinnamon
- 2 tablespoons honey or maple syrup (optional)
- Fresh fruit slices (e.g., bananas, strawberries) for topping

Nutritional Information: Calories: 180 | Protein: 4g | Carbohydrates: 38g | Fat: 2g | Fiber: 1g

Instructions:

1. Wash the white rice under cold water until the rinse water becomes clear.
2. After rinsing the rice, transfer it to a medium saucepan and add the water.
3. Bring to a boil, then reduce heat to low, cover, and simmer for 12-15 minutes or until the rice is tender and most of the water is absorbed.
4. Stir in the almond milk, ground cinnamon, and honey or maple syrup if using. Cook for an additional 3-5 minutes, stirring occasionally, until the mixture thickens to your desired consistency.
5. Remove from heat and let it sit for a minute to cool slightly.

6. Divide the warm rice cereal into bowls and top with fresh fruit slices.

7. Serve immediately and enjoy the comforting warmth and sweetness of this cinnamon-spiced rice cereal.

Serving Suggestions:

- Top with sliced bananas, a drizzle of honey or maple syrup, and a sprinkle of chopped nuts for crunch.

Jicama Toast

- **Preparation Time:** 10 minutes
- **Serves:** 4

Ingredients:

- 1 large jicama, peeled and sliced into 1/4-inch thick rounds
- 2 tablespoons olive oil
- 1/4 teaspoon salt
- 1/4 teaspoon black pepper

Nutritional Information: (per serving without toppings): Calories: 90, Carbs: 16g, Fiber: 9g, Protein: 1g, Fat: 3g

Instructions:

1. Peel the jicama and slice it into 1/4-inch thick rounds using a sharp knife or a mandoline slicer.

2. Arrange the jicama slices on a baking sheet or plate.

3. Brush the jicama slices with olive oil on both sides, or lightly spray with cooking oil.

4. Sprinkle with salt and black pepper.

5. Toast the jicama slices in a preheated oven or toaster oven at 400°F (200°C) for about 5-7 minutes, or until lightly browned and slightly crispy. Be careful not to overcook, as they can turn dry and tough.

6. Remove from the oven and let cool slightly before adding your desired toppings.

Serving Suggestions:

- Top it with avocado, nut butter, sliced hard-boiled eggs, smoked salmon, or any other protein-rich topping of your choice.

Scrambled Eggs with Spinach and Feta

- **Preparation Time:** 15 minutes
- **Serves:** 2

Ingredients:

- 4 large eggs
- 1 cup fresh spinach leaves, chopped
- 1/4 cup crumbled feta cheese
- 1 tablespoon olive oil
- Salt and pepper to taste

Nutritional Information: Calories: 240 | Protein: 16g | Carbohydrates: 3g | Fat: 19g | Fiber: 1g

Instructions:

1. Crack the eggs into a bowl and whisk until well beaten. Season with salt and pepper.
2. Heat olive oil in a non-stick skillet over medium heat.

3. Add chopped spinach to the skillet and sauté until wilted.

4. Pour the beaten eggs into the skillet with the spinach.

5. Using a spatula, gently scramble the eggs and spinach mixture until the eggs are cooked through but still moist.

6. Sprinkle crumbled feta cheese over the scrambled eggs and stir briefly to combine.

7. Remove from heat and transfer the scrambled eggs to a plate.

8. Serve the Scrambled Eggs with Spinach and Feta hot, garnished with fresh herbs if desired.

Serving Suggestions:

- Serve alongside whole-grain toast or a toasted English muffin.
- For a touch of fresh color and vibrancy, garnish with parsley or chives.

Papaya "Boats" with Chia Pudding

- **Preparation Time:** 20 minutes (plus chilling time for chia pudding)
- **Serves:** 2

Ingredients:

For Chia Pudding:

- 1/4 cup chia seeds
- 1 cup almond milk
- 1 tablespoon honey or maple syrup (optional)
- 1/2 teaspoon vanilla extract

For Papaya "Boats":

- 1 ripe papaya, halved and seeds removed
- Fresh berries (e.g., strawberries, blueberries) for topping
- Fresh mint leaves for garnish

Nutritional Information: Chia Pudding - Per Serving (without sweetener): Calories: 120 | Protein: 4g | Carbohydrates: 11g | Fat: 7g | Fiber: 9g

Instructions:

1. In a bowl, combine chia seeds, almond milk, honey or maple syrup (if using), and vanilla extract. Stir well to combine.

2. Cover the bowl and refrigerate for at least 2 hours or overnight, allowing the chia seeds to absorb the liquid and form a pudding-like consistency.

3. Once the chia pudding is ready, scoop it into the hollowed-out papaya halves, creating "boats."

4. Top the chia pudding-filled papaya boats with fresh berries of your choice.

5. Garnish with fresh mint leaves for added freshness and presentation.

6. Serve the Papaya "Boats" with Chia Pudding chilled and enjoy the delightful combination of creamy chia pudding and juicy papaya.

Serving Suggestions:

- Serve with a side of Greek yogurt for extra creaminess.

Melon and Cottage Cheese Medley

- **Preparation Time:** 10 minutes
- **Serves:** 2

Ingredients:

- 1 cup diced honeydew melon
- 1 cup diced cantaloupe melon
- 1/2 cup low-fat cottage cheese
- 2 tablespoons honey or agave syrup (optional)
- Fresh mint leaves for garnish

Nutritional Information: Calories: 150 | Protein: 8g | Carbohydrates: 30g | Fat: 1g | Fiber: 2g

Instructions:

1. In a mixing bowl, combine the diced honeydew and cantaloupe melons.
2. Spoon the low-fat cottage cheese over the melon mixture.
3. Drizzle honey or agave syrup over the melon and cottage cheese.

4. Gently toss the ingredients together to coat the melons with the sweetened cottage cheese.

5. Divide the Melon and Cottage Cheese Medley into serving bowls.

6. Serve the medley immediately and enjoy the juicy sweetness of the melons paired with creamy cottage cheese.

Serving Suggestions:

- Garnish with fresh mint leaves and a drizzle of honey for added sweetness.

- Enjoy with a slice of whole-grain toast.

Poached Pears with Vanilla Bean Ricotta

- **Preparation Time:** 30 minutes
- **Serves:** 2

Ingredients:

- 2 ripe pears, peeled and halved
- 2 cups water
- 1/4 cup honey
- 1 vanilla bean pod (or 1 teaspoon vanilla extract)
- 1/2 cup ricotta cheese

- 1 tablespoon powdered sugar (optional)
- Fresh berries for garnish

Nutritional Information: Calories: 250 | Protein: 8g | Carbohydrates: 50g | Fat: 4g | Fiber: 6g

Instructions:

1. In a saucepan, combine water, honey, and the seeds scraped from the vanilla bean pod (or vanilla extract).
2. Gently simmer the mixture over medium heat, achieving small bubbles around the edges.
3. Add the peeled and halved pears to the simmering liquid, ensuring they are submerged.
4. Poach the pears for about 15-20 minutes or until tender when pierced with a fork.
5. Remove the poached pears from the liquid and let them cool slightly.
6. In a small bowl, mix the ricotta cheese with powdered sugar (if using) until smooth.
7. To serve, place a dollop of vanilla bean ricotta on each poached pear half.

8. Garnish with fresh berries and a drizzle of the poaching liquid.

9. Serve the Poached Pears with Vanilla Bean Ricotta warm or chilled, enjoying the delicate sweetness and creamy richness.

Serving Suggestions:

- Pair it with a slice of toasted brioche or whole-grain bread for a delightful contrast of textures.

Lunch Recipes for Gastroparesis Diet Miso Soup with Silken Tofu and Seaweed

- **Preparation Time:** 15 minutes
- **Serves:** 4

Ingredients:

- 4 cups water
- 4 tablespoons miso paste
- 1 cup silken tofu, cubed
- 2 tablespoons dried wakame seaweed
- 2 green onions, thinly sliced
- 1 tablespoon soy sauce (optional)

- Dash of sesame oil (optional)

Nutritional Information: Calories: 70 | Protein: 4g | Carbohydrates: 5g | Fat: 3g | Fiber: 1g

Instructions:

1. In a medium pot, bring water to a gentle simmer over medium heat.

2. In a small bowl, dissolve miso paste in a ladleful of hot water from the pot, then add it back to the pot.

3. Add cubed silken tofu and dried wakame seaweed to the pot. Simmer gently for 5-7 minutes.

4. Stir in sliced green onions and soy sauce (if using). Cook for another 1-2 minutes.

5. Remove the pot from heat and add a dash of sesame oil (if using) for extra flavor.

6. Serve the Miso Soup with Silken Tofu and Seaweed hot in bowls.

7. Garnish with additional green onions or a sprinkle of sesame seeds for presentation.

Serving Suggestions:

- Pair it with steamed rice or a side of mixed greens dressed in a light vinaigrette for a complete and satisfying lunch experience.

Chicken Lettuce Wraps with Low-Sodium Soy Sauce

- **Preparation Time:** 25 minutes
- **Serves:** 4

Ingredients:

- 1 lb ground chicken breast
- 1 tablespoon sesame oil
- 2 cloves garlic, minced
- 1 tablespoon grated fresh ginger
- 1/4 cup low-sodium soy sauce
- 1 tablespoon rice vinegar
- 1 teaspoon Sriracha sauce (optional, for a little heat)
- 1 cup shredded carrots
- 1/2 cup sliced green onions
- 8-10 large lettuce leaves (Bibb, Boston, or Iceberg)

Nutritional Information: Calories: 210, Carbs: 6g, Fiber: 2g, Protein: 26g, Fat: 9g

Instructions:

1. In a large skillet or wok, heat the sesame oil over medium-high heat.

2. Add the ground chicken, garlic, and grated ginger. Cook, breaking up the chicken with a wooden spoon, until no longer pink, about 5-7 minutes.
3. Add the low-sodium soy sauce, rice vinegar, and Sriracha sauce (if using). Stir to combine.
4. Remove from heat and stir in the shredded carrots and sliced green onions.
5. To serve, spoon the chicken mixture into lettuce leaves and enjoy like a taco or wrap.

Serving Suggestions:

- Serve them with additional sliced vegetables like cucumber or radish for added crunch and fiber. You can also pair them with a small portion of cooked quinoa or brown rice for additional nutrients.

Zucchini Noodles with Pesto

- **Preparation Time:** 20 minutes
- **Serves:** 2

Ingredients:

- 2 medium zucchinis
- 1 cup fresh basil leaves
- 1/4 cup pine nuts

- 1/4 cup grated Parmesan cheese
- 2 cloves garlic
- 1/4 cup olive oil
- Salt and pepper to taste
- Cherry tomatoes (for garnish)
- Fresh basil leaves (for garnish)

Nutritional Information: Calories: 250 | Protein: 7g | Carbohydrates: 10g | Fat: 21g | Fiber: 4g

Instructions:

1. Using a spiralizer, spiralize the zucchinis into noodles. Set aside.

2. In a food processor, combine basil leaves, pine nuts, grated Parmesan cheese, garlic, and olive oil. Blend until smooth and creamy.

3. Give the pesto a taste and adjust the seasoning with salt and pepper as desired

4. Heat a large skillet over medium heat. Add the zucchini noodles and cook for 2-3 minutes until just tender.

5. Add the pesto sauce to the skillet with the zucchini noodles. Toss gently to coat the noodles evenly with the sauce.

6. Cook for another minute to heat through.

7. Remove from heat and divide the Zucchini Noodles with Pesto into serving bowls.

8. Garnish with halved cherry tomatoes and fresh basil leaves.

9. Serve immediately, enjoying the vibrant flavors and freshness of the zucchini noodles with pesto.

Serving Suggestions:

- Pair with grilled chicken or shrimp for added protein.

- Enjoy with a side of garlic bread or a mixed green salad for a complete and delicious meal.

Tuna Salad on Endive Spears

- **Preparation Time:** 15 minutes

- **Serves:** 4

Ingredients:

- 2 cans (5 ounces each) tuna, drained

- 1/4 cup mayonnaise

- 1 tablespoon Dijon mustard

- 2 tablespoons chopped red onion

- 1/4 cup diced celery

- Salt and pepper to taste
- Endive spears (for serving)
- Cherry tomatoes (for garnish)
- Fresh parsley (for garnish)

Nutritional Information: Calories: 180 | Protein: 20g | Carbohydrates: 2g | Fat: 10g | Fiber: 1g

Instructions:

1. In a mixing bowl, combine drained tuna, mayonnaise, Dijon mustard, chopped red onion, and diced celery. Mix well to combine.
2. Season the tuna salad with salt and pepper to taste.
3. Arrange endive spears on a serving platter.
4. Spoon the tuna salad onto each endive spear, creating appetizing bites.
5. Garnish with halved cherry tomatoes and fresh parsley leaves.
6. Serve the Tuna Salad on Endive Spears chilled or at room temperature.

Serving Suggestions:

- Pair with a side of whole-grain crackers or crusty bread for added texture.

Poached Salmon with Roasted Asparagus and Lemon

- **Preparation Time:** 30 minutes
- **Serves:** 2

Ingredients:

- 2 salmon filets
- Salt and pepper to taste
- 1 bunch asparagus, trimmed
- 2 tablespoons olive oil
- 1 lemon, thinly sliced
- Fresh dill (for garnish)

Nutritional Information: Calories: 350 | Protein: 35g | Carbohydrates: 6g | Fat: 21g | Fiber: 3g

Instructions:

1. Preheat your oven to 400°F (200°C).
2. Season the salmon filets with salt and pepper to taste.

3. Arrange the trimmed asparagus on a baking sheet and drizzle with olive oil. Season with salt and pepper.

4. Place the seasoned salmon filets on the same baking sheet, skin-side down.

5. Top the salmon filets with thinly sliced lemon rounds.

6. Roast in the preheated oven for 15-20 minutes or until the salmon is cooked through and flakes easily with a fork.

7. Remove from the oven and let it rest for a few minutes, garnish with fresh dill before serving.

Serving Suggestions:

- Pair with a side of quinoa or wild rice for added fiber and nutrients.

Pureed Broccoli and Cheddar Soup with Low-Fat Crackers

- **Preparation Time:** 30 minutes
- **Serves:** 4

Ingredients:

- 1 head broccoli, chopped

- 1 onion, chopped
- 2 cloves garlic, minced
- 4 cups low-sodium vegetable broth
- 1 cup low-fat milk
- 1 cup shredded low-fat cheddar cheese
- Salt and pepper to taste
- Low-fat crackers (for serving)
- Fresh parsley (for garnish)

Nutritional Information: Calories: 150 | Protein: 10g | Carbohydrates: 15g | Fat: 6g | Fiber: 5g

Instructions:

1. In a large pot, heat a little olive oil over medium heat.
2. Add chopped onion and minced garlic to the pot, sauté until softened and fragrant.
3. Add chopped broccoli to the pot and sauté for a few minutes.
4. Pour in low-sodium vegetable broth and bring to a boil, reduce heat and simmer until the broccoli is tender.
5. Use an immersion blender or transfer the mixture to a blender to puree until smooth.

6. Return the pureed soup to the pot over low heat.

7. Stir in low-fat milk and shredded low-fat cheddar cheese until the cheese is melted and incorporated.

8. Season with salt and pepper to taste.

9. Serve the Pureed Broccoli and Cheddar Soup hot, garnished with fresh parsley.

10. Serve with low-fat crackers on the side.

Serving Suggestions:

- Pair with a side salad of mixed greens dressed in a light vinaigrette for added freshness.

Shrimp Skewers with Roasted Bell Peppers and Couscous

- **Preparation Time:** 30 minutes (plus marinating time)
- **Serves:** 2

Ingredients:

- 10-12 large shrimp, peeled and deveined
- 1 red bell pepper, chopped into bite-sized pieces
- 1 yellow bell pepper, cut into chunks
- 2 tablespoons olive oil
- 2 cloves garlic, minced

- 1 teaspoon paprika
- Salt and pepper to taste
- 1 cup couscous
- Fresh parsley (for garnish)

Nutritional Information: Calories: 350 | Protein: 25g | Carbohydrates: 35g | Fat: 12g | Fiber: 4g

Instructions:

1. In a bowl, combine olive oil, minced garlic, paprika, salt, and pepper. Toss the peeled and deveined shrimp in the marinade to absorb delicious flavors. Let them marinate for 15-20 minutes.

2. Preheat your grill or grill pan to medium-high heat in preparation for cooking.

3. Thread the marinated shrimp on skewers, alternating with chunks of red and yellow bell peppers.

4. Grill the shrimp skewers for 2-3 minutes per side or until the shrimp is cooked through and lightly charred.

5. While the shrimp is grilling, prepare the couscous according to the package instructions.

6. Once the couscous is cooked, fluff it with a fork and divide it onto serving plates.

7. Place the grilled shrimp skewers and roasted bell peppers on top of the couscous.

8. Garnish with fresh parsley before serving.

Serving Suggestions:

- Pair with a side of tzatziki sauce or a dollop of hummus for added creaminess and flavor.

Dinner Recipes for Diabetic Gastroparesis Diet

Turkey Meatballs with Pureed Vegetables and Mashed Cauliflower

- **Preparation Time:** 50 minutes
- **Serves:** 4

Ingredients:

For the Turkey Meatballs:

- 1 lb ground turkey breast
- 1 egg
- 1/4 cup almond flour
- 1/4 cup grated Parmesan cheese

- 1 teaspoon dried basil
- 1 teaspoon dried oregano
- 1/2 teaspoon salt
- 1/4 teaspoon black pepper

For the Pureed Vegetables:
- 1 cup diced carrots
- 1 cup diced zucchini
- 1/2 cup diced onion
- 2 cloves garlic, minced
- 1 cup low-sodium vegetable broth

For the Mashed Cauliflower:
- 1 head cauliflower, cut into florets
- 2 tablespoons olive oil
- 1/4 cup unsweetened almond milk
- Salt and pepper to taste

Nutritional Information: Calories: 330, Carbs: 16g, Fiber: 6g, Protein: 30g, Fat: 18g

Instructions:
1. Preheat oven to 400°F (200°C).
2. In a large bowl, combine all ingredients for the turkey meatballs and mix well.

3. Form the mixture into small meatballs, about 1-inch in size, and place them on a baking sheet lined with parchment paper.

4. Bake the meatballs for 18-20 minutes, or until fully cooked through.

5. While the meatballs are baking, prepare the pureed vegetables by sautéing the carrots, zucchini, onion, and garlic in a skillet with a little olive oil or cooking spray until softened.

6. Transfer the sautéed vegetables to a blender or food processor, add the vegetable broth, and puree until smooth.

7. To make the mashed cauliflower, steam or boil the cauliflower florets until tender.

8. Drain the cauliflower and transfer it to a food processor or blender.

9. Add olive oil, almond milk, salt, and pepper, and puree until smooth and creamy.

10. Serve the turkey meatballs over a bed of pureed vegetables, with a side of mashed cauliflower.

Serving Suggestions:

- You can garnish with fresh herbs like parsley or chives for added flavor. Serve with a side salad or roasted non-starchy vegetables for extra fiber and nutrients.

Baked Tilapia Caesar Salad with Low-Fat Dressing

- **Preparation Time:** 30 minutes
- **Serves:** 2

Ingredients:

- 2 tilapia filets
- Salt and pepper to taste
- 1 tablespoon olive oil
- 4 cups chopped romaine lettuce
- 1/4 cup grated Parmesan cheese
- Whole-grain croutons (optional)

- Low-fat Caesar dressing (store-bought or homemade)
- Lemon wedges (for garnish)

Nutritional Information: Calories: 250 | Protein: 30g | Carbohydrates: 10g | Fat: 10g | Fiber: 3g

Instructions:

1. Preheat your oven to 375°F (190°C).
2. Season tilapia filets with salt and pepper on both sides.
3. Heat olive oil in an oven-safe skillet over medium-high heat, add tilapia filets to the skillet and sear for 2-3 minutes on each side until golden brown.
4. Transfer the skillet to the preheated oven and bake the tilapia for 10-12 minutes until cooked through.
5. While the tilapia is baking, prepare the salad by combining chopped romaine lettuce and grated Parmesan cheese in a large bowl.
6. Add whole-grain croutons (if using) to the salad.
7. Drizzle low-fat Caesar dressing over the salad and toss to coat evenly.

8. Once the tilapia is done baking, remove it from the oven and let it rest for a few minutes.

9. Divide the Caesar salad onto serving plates and top each serving with a baked tilapia filet.

10. Garnish with lemon wedges for added flavor.

Serving Suggestions:

- Pair with a side of steamed broccoli or grilled vegetables for added nutrients and texture.

Lentil Soup with Low-Fat Vegetable Broth

- **Preparation Time:** 45 minutes
- **Serves:** 4

Ingredients:

- 1 cup of dried lentils, rinsed clean and drained thoroughly
- 4 cups low-fat vegetable broth
- 1 onion, chopped
- 2 carrots, diced
- 2 celery stalks, diced
- 2 cloves garlic, minced
- 1 teaspoon dried thyme

- 1 teaspoon dried oregano
- Salt and pepper to taste
- Fresh parsley (for garnish)
- Lemon wedges (for serving)

Nutritional Information: Calories: 200 | Protein: 15g | Carbohydrates: 35g | Fat: 1g | Fiber: 12g

Instructions:

1. In a large pot, combine rinsed lentils, low-fat vegetable broth, chopped onion, diced carrots, diced celery, minced garlic, dried thyme, and dried oregano.

2. Heat the mixture over medium-high heat, bringing it to a full boil.

3. Reduce heat to low, cover the pot, and simmer the lentil soup for 30-35 minutes or until the lentils and vegetables are tender.

4. Give the soup a taste and adjust the seasoning with salt and pepper as desired.

5. Take the pot off the heat and allow the soup to cool down a bit before proceeding.

6. Use an immersion blender or transfer a portion of the soup to a blender to puree until smooth (optional for a creamier texture).

7. Ladle the Lentil Soup with Low-Fat Vegetable Broth into serving bowls.

8. Garnish with fresh parsley and serve with lemon wedges on the side for squeezing over the soup.

Serving Suggestions:

- Pair with a slice of whole-grain bread or a side of quinoa for added fiber and carbohydrates.

Grilled Lean Beef Tenderloin with Garlic Spinach Purée

- **Preparation Time:** 40 minutes
- **Serves:** 4

Ingredients:

For the Beef Tenderloin:

- 1 lb beef tenderloin, trimmed
- 2 tablespoons olive oil
- 1 teaspoon dried thyme
- 1 teaspoon dried rosemary
- Salt and pepper to taste

For the Garlic Spinach Purée:

- 1 lb fresh spinach leaves
- 2 cloves garlic, minced
- 2 tablespoons olive oil
- 1/4 cup unsweetened almond milk
- Salt and pepper to taste

Nutritional Information: Calories: 315, Carbs: 5g, Fiber: 2g, Protein: 34g, Fat: 20g

Instructions:

1. Preheat an outdoor grill or indoor grill pan to medium-high heat.
2. Rub the beef tenderloin with olive oil, thyme, rosemary, salt, and pepper.
3. Grill the tenderloin for 20-25 minutes, turning occasionally, until it reaches the desired doneness (145°F for medium-rare).
4. While the beef is grilling, prepare the garlic spinach purée by sautéing the minced garlic in olive oil for 1 minute.
5. Add the fresh spinach leaves and continue to sauté until the spinach is wilted, about 2-3 minutes.
6. Transfer the spinach mixture to a blender or food processor, add the almond milk, salt, and pepper.
7. Purée until smooth and creamy.
8. Once the tenderloin is cooked, transfer it to a cutting board and let it rest for 5 minutes before slicing.

9. Serve the sliced beef tenderloin with the garlic spinach purée on the side.

Serving Suggestions:

- Serve with a side salad or roasted non-starchy vegetables for added nutrients. You can also garnish the dish with fresh herbs like parsley or chives for extra flavor.

Beef Stew with Pureed Vegetables and Cauliflower Breadsticks

- **Preparation Time:** 2 hours 20 minutes
- **Serves:** 4

Ingredients:

For the Beef Stew:

- 1 lb lean beef stew meat, cut into 1-inch cubes
- 2 tablespoons olive oil
- 1 onion, diced
- 3 cloves garlic, minced
- 2 cups low-sodium beef broth
- 2 carrots, peeled and diced
- 2 celery stalks, diced

- 1 bay leaf
- 1 teaspoon dried thyme
- Salt and pepper to taste

For the Pureed Vegetables:

- 1 cup diced zucchini
- 1 cup diced bell pepper
- 1 cup low-sodium vegetable broth

For the Cauliflower Breadsticks:

- 1 head cauliflower, cut into florets
- 2 eggs
- 1/2 cup almond flour
- 1/4 cup grated Parmesan cheese
- 1 teaspoon dried Italian seasoning
- Salt and pepper to taste

Nutritional Information: Calories: 410, Carbs: 18g, Fiber: 6g, Protein: 36g, Fat: 22g

Instructions:

1. In a Dutch oven or large pot, warm the olive oil over medium-high heat.
2. Add the beef cubes and brown them on all sides, about 5 minutes.

3. Add the onion and garlic, and sauté for 2-3 minutes until fragrant.

4. Pour in the beef broth, and add the carrots, celery, bay leaf, thyme, salt, and pepper.

5. Bring the stew to a boil, then reduce the heat to low, cover, and simmer for 1.5 hours.

6. While the stew is simmering, prepare the pureed vegetables by sautéing the zucchini and bell pepper until softened.

7. Transfer the sautéed vegetables to a blender or food processor, add the vegetable broth, and puree until smooth.

8. To make the cauliflower breadsticks, steam or boil the cauliflower florets until tender.

9. Drain the cauliflower and transfer it to a food processor or blender, along with the eggs, almond flour, Parmesan cheese, Italian seasoning, salt, and pepper.

10. Pulse the mixture until it forms a dough-like consistency.

11. Roll the dough into long breadstick shapes and place them on a baking sheet lined with parchment paper.

12. Bake the breadsticks at 400°F (200°C) for 15-20 minutes, or until golden brown.

13. Serve the beef stew over a bed of pureed vegetables, with cauliflower breadsticks on the side.

Serving Suggestions:

- Serve with a side salad or roasted non-starchy vegetables for added fiber and nutrients.

Baked Cod with Lemon Butter Sauce and Quinoa

- **Preparation Time:** 30 minutes
- **Serves:** 2

Ingredients:

- 2 cod filets
- Salt and pepper to taste
- 2 tablespoons olive oil
- 2 tablespoons unsalted butter
- 2 cloves garlic, minced
- Juice of 1 lemon

- 1 tablespoon chopped fresh parsley
- 1 cup cooked quinoa
- Lemon wedges (for serving)

Nutritional Information: Calories: 300 | Protein: 30g | Carbohydrates: 15g | Fat: 15g | Fiber: 2g

Instructions:

1. Preheat your oven to 400°F (200°C), grease a baking dish with olive oil.
2. Season cod filets with salt and pepper on both sides.
3. Place the seasoned cod filets in the greased baking dish.
4. In a small saucepan, heat olive oil and unsalted butter over medium heat until the butter is melted.
5. Add minced garlic to the saucepan and sauté for 1-2 minutes until fragrant.
6. Remove the saucepan from heat and stir in lemon juice and chopped fresh parsley.
7. Pour the lemon butter sauce over the cod filets in the baking dish.
8. Bake the cod in the preheated oven for 15-20 minutes or until the fish is cooked through and flakes easily with a fork.
9. While the cod is baking, prepare quinoa according to package instructions.
10. Serve the Baked Cod with Lemon Butter Sauce hot, accompanied by cooked quinoa and lemon wedges for squeezing over the fish.

Serving Suggestions:

- Pair with a side of steamed broccoli or asparagus for added fiber and nutrients.

Steamed Fish Fillet with Grilled Portobello Mushroom Caps

- **Preparation Time:** 30 minutes
- **Serves:** 2

Ingredients:

- 2 fish filets (such as tilapia, cod, or salmon)
- Salt and pepper to taste
- 2 tablespoons olive oil
- 2 portobello mushroom caps
- 2 cloves garlic, minced
- 1 tablespoon balsamic vinegar
- Fresh parsley (for garnish)
- Lemon wedges (for serving)

Nutritional Information: Calories: 250 | Protein: 30g | Carbohydrates: 10g | Fat: 12g | Fiber: 4g

Instructions:

1. Sprinkle both sides of the fish fillets with salt and pepper.

2. Heat olive oil in a skillet over medium-high heat, add fish filets to the skillet and cook for 3-4 minutes per side or until cooked through and flaky.

3. Remove the fish filets from the skillet and set aside.

4. In the same skillet, add minced garlic and sauté until fragrant.

5. Add portobello mushroom caps to the skillet and cook for 3-4 minutes per side until tender.

6. Drizzle balsamic vinegar over the mushroom caps and cook for another minute.

7. Remove the mushroom caps from the skillet and set aside.

8. Arrange the steamed fish filets on a serving platter.

9. Place grilled portobello mushroom caps on top of the fish filets.

10. Garnish with fresh parsley and serve with lemon wedges on the side.

Serving Suggestions:

- Garnish with fresh parsley and serve with lemon wedges on the side for squeezing over the fish.

Desserts and Snacks for Gastroparesis Diet

Avocado Chocolate Mousse

- **Preparation Time:** 15 minutes
- **Serves:** 2

Ingredients:

- 1 ripe avocado
- 2 tablespoons unsweetened cocoa powder
- 2 tablespoons honey or maple syrup
- 1 teaspoon vanilla extract
- Pinch of salt
- 1/4 cup almond milk or any preferred milk alternative
- Dark chocolate shavings or cocoa powder for garnish (optional)

Nutritional Information: Calories: 200 | Protein: 3g | Carbohydrates: 20g | Fat: 14g | Fiber: 7g

Instructions:

1. Cut the ripe avocado in half, remove the pit, and scoop out the flesh into a blender or food processor.

2. Add unsweetened cocoa powder, honey or maple syrup, vanilla extract, pinch of salt, and almond milk to the blender.

3. Blend all the ingredients until smooth and creamy, scraping down the sides of the blender as needed.

4. Taste the mousse and adjust sweetness or cocoa flavor if desired.

5. Scoop the avocado chocolate mousse to serving bowls or glasses.

6. Chill the mousse in the refrigerator for at least 30 minutes to allow it to set and enhance the flavor.

7. Before serving, garnish with dark chocolate shavings or a sprinkle of cocoa powder for added visual appeal.

Serving Suggestions:

- Top with fresh berries or a dollop of whipped cream for added sweetness and texture.

Homemade Applesauce

- **Preparation Time:** 30 minutes
- **Serves:** 4

Ingredients:

- 4 medium-sized apples (such as Granny Smith or Fuji), peeled, cored, and chopped
- 1/2 cup water
- 2 tablespoons honey or maple syrup (optional)
- 1 teaspoon ground cinnamon (optional)

Nutritional Information: Calories: 80 | Protein: 0g | Carbohydrates: 20g | Fat: 0g | Fiber: 3g

Instructions:

1. In a saucepan, combine chopped apples, water, honey or maple syrup (if using), and ground cinnamon (if using), bring the mixture to a boil over medium heat.

2. Reduce heat to low, cover the saucepan, and simmer the apples for about 20-25 minutes or until they are soft and tender.

3. Remove the saucepan from heat and let the applesauce cool slightly.

4. Use a potato masher or immersion blender to puree the cooked apples until smooth (adjust the consistency by adding more water if needed).

5. Taste the applesauce and add more honey, maple syrup, or cinnamon to suit your preference.

6. Transfer the homemade applesauce to a serving bowl or jar.

7. Serve the applesauce warm or chilled, depending on your preference.

Serving Suggestions:

- Sprinkle it with a dash of cinnamon or nutmeg for extra flavor.

Mango Sorbet

- **Preparation Time:** 10 minutes (plus freezing time)
- **Serves:** 4

Ingredients:

- 2 ripe mangoes, peeled, pitted, and chopped
- 2 tablespoons honey or agave syrup (optional, depending on the sweetness of mangoes)
- Juice of 1 lime
- 1/4 cup water

Nutritional Information: Calories: 90 | Protein: 1g | Carbohydrates: 23g | Fat: 0g | Fiber: 2g

Instructions:

1. Place the chopped mangoes, honey or agave syrup (if using), lime juice, and water in a blender or food processor.

2. Blend the ingredients until smooth and completely combined.

3. Taste the mixture and adjust sweetness by adding more honey or agave syrup if needed.

4. Pour the mango mixture into a shallow, freezer-safe container.

5. Cover the container with a lid or plastic wrap and place it in the freezer.

6. Freeze the mango mixture for at least 4-6 hours or until firm, stirring every hour to prevent ice crystals from forming.

7. Once the mango sorbet is frozen and firm, remove it from the freezer and let it sit at room temperature for a few minutes to soften slightly.

8. Scoop the mango sorbet into serving bowls or cones.

9. Garnish with fresh mint leaves or sliced mangoes for an extra touch.

Serving Suggestions:

- Enjoy it on its own or pair it with fresh fruit slices, such as strawberries or kiwi, for a colorful and delicious presentation.

Lemon Coconut Energy Bites

- **Preparation Time:** 1 hour 15 minutes (plus chilling time)
- **Serves:** 12 bites

Ingredients:

- 1 cup unsweetened shredded coconut
- 1/2 cup almond flour
- 1/4 cup coconut oil, melted
- 2 tablespoons lemon juice
- 1 tablespoon lemon zest
- 2 tablespoons monk fruit sweetener or erythritol (or stevia to taste)

Nutritional Information (per bite): Calories: 110, Carbs: 4g, Fiber: 2g, Protein: 2g, Fat: 10g

Instructions:

1. In a medium bowl, mix together the shredded coconut, almond flour, melted coconut oil, lemon juice, lemon zest, and monk fruit sweetener/erythritol until well combined.
2. Shape the mixture into small balls, approximately 1 inch in diameter.

3. Place the energy bites on a parchment-lined baking sheet or plate.

4. Chill the formed balls in the refrigerator for at least 1 hour, or until they become firm.

5. Store the energy bites in an airtight container in the refrigerator for up to 1 week.

Serving Suggestions:

- Enjoy them as a grab-and-go snack or as a light dessert option.

Pumpkin Custard

- **Preparation Time:** 40 minutes
- **Serves:** 4

Ingredients:

- 1 cup canned pumpkin puree
- 1/2 cup coconut milk (or any preferred milk)
- 2 large eggs
- 1/4 cup honey or maple syrup
- 1 teaspoon vanilla extract
- 1 teaspoon ground cinnamon

- 1/4 teaspoon ground nutmeg
- Pinch of salt
- Whipped cream or coconut whipped cream (optional, for serving)
- Ground cinnamon or nutmeg, for garnish (optional)

Nutritional Information: Calories: 150 | Protein: 5g | Carbohydrates: 20g | Fat: 6g | Fiber: 3g

Instructions:

1. Preheat your oven to 350°F (175°C) and grease four ramekins or custard cups.
2. In a mixing bowl, combine pumpkin puree, coconut milk, eggs, honey or maple syrup, vanilla extract, ground cinnamon, ground nutmeg, and a pinch of salt.
3. Whisk all the ingredients together until smooth and well combined.
4. Pour the pumpkin custard mixture evenly into the greased ramekins or custard cups.

5. Place the ramekins in a baking dish and fill the dish with enough hot water to reach halfway up the sides of the ramekins (this creates a water bath).

6. Carefully transfer the baking dish to the preheated oven and bake the custards for 25-30 minutes or until set but still slightly jiggly in the center.

7. Remove the baking dish from the oven and let the custards cool to room temperature.

8. Once cooled, cover the ramekins with plastic wrap and refrigerate the custards for at least 2 hours or until chilled and firm.

9. Before serving, top each pumpkin custard with a dollop of whipped cream or coconut whipped cream (if using) and a sprinkle of ground cinnamon or nutmeg for garnish.

Serving Suggestions:

- Garnish with a drizzle of caramel sauce or a sprinkle of chopped nuts for added indulgence.

Beverages/Drinks for Gastroparesis Diet

Lemon Ginger Elixir

- **Preparation Time:** 10 minutes
- **Serves:** 2

Ingredients:

- 2 cups water
- 1-inch fresh ginger root, peeled and thinly sliced
- 1 lemon, juiced
- 2 tablespoons honey or maple syrup (optional)
- Fresh mint leaves for garnish (optional)

Nutritional Information: Calories: 20 | Carbohydrates: 5g | Sugars: 3g | Vitamin C: 20% DV

Instructions:

1. In a small saucepan, bring 2 cups of water to a gentle boil.

2. Add the thinly sliced fresh ginger to the boiling water.

3. Reduce the heat and let the ginger simmer in the water for about 5-7 minutes to infuse its flavor.

4. Remove the saucepan from heat and let the ginger water cool slightly.

5. Strain the ginger water into a pitcher or glass to remove the ginger slices.

6. Add freshly squeezed lemon juice to the ginger water and stir well.

7. Taste the elixir and add honey or maple syrup if you prefer a sweeter taste, stirring until dissolved.

8. Pour the Lemon Ginger Elixir into serving glasses.

9. Garnish with fresh mint leaves for a refreshing touch.

Serving Suggestions:

- Pair with a slice of lemon or a sprig of mint for an aesthetically pleasing presentation.

Pomegranate Juice

- **Preparation Time:** 10 minutes
- **Serves:** 2

Ingredients:

- 2 large pomegranates
- 1/2 cup water
- 1 tablespoon honey or agave syrup (optional, for sweetness)

Nutritional Information: Calories: 80 | Carbohydrates: 20g | Sugars: 15g | Vitamin C: 15% DV | Antioxidants: High

Instructions:

1. Cut the pomegranates in half and extract the seeds, discarding any white membranes.
2. Place the pomegranate seeds in a blender or juicer.
3. Add water to the blender or juicer to help with blending.

4. Blend or juice the pomegranate seeds until smooth and well combined.

5. Strain the pomegranate juice through a fine-mesh sieve or cheesecloth to remove any pulp.

6. Add honey or agave syrup to the strained juice if desired, stirring until dissolved.

7. Pour the Pomegranate Juice into serving glasses.

8. Serve chilled with ice cubes or garnish with a few pomegranate arils for decoration.

Serving Suggestions:

- Garnish with a few pomegranate arils or a slice of lime for a decorative touch.

Unsweetened Golden Milk

- **Preparation Time:** 25 minutes
- **Serves:** 2

Ingredients:

- 2 cups unsweetened almond milk (or any preferred milk)

- 1 teaspoon ground turmeric
- 1/2 teaspoon ground cinnamon
- 1/4 teaspoon ground ginger
- Pinch of black pepper
- Pinch of ground cardamom (optional)
- Pinch of ground nutmeg (optional)
- Honey or maple syrup (optional, for sweetness)

Nutritional Information: Calories: 30 | Carbohydrates: 2g | Fat: 2g | Fiber: 1g | Vitamin D: 25% DV

Instructions:

1. In a small saucepan, heat the unsweetened almond milk over medium heat until warmed but not boiling.
2. Add ground turmeric, ground cinnamon, ground ginger, black pepper, and any optional spices like ground cardamom and nutmeg to the warm almond milk.
3. Whisk the ingredients together until the spices are well dissolved and the milk is infused with golden color.

4. Simmer the golden milk mixture for about 5 minutes, stirring occasionally.

5. Remove the saucepan from heat and let the golden milk cool slightly.

6. Taste the golden milk and add honey or maple syrup if desired for sweetness, stirring until dissolved.

7. Pour the Unsweetened Golden Milk into serving cups or mugs.

8. Serve warm and enjoy the comforting and anti-inflammatory benefits of this nourishing beverage.

Serving Suggestions:

- Garnish with a sprinkle of ground cinnamon or a cinnamon stick for added flavor and aroma.

Chamomile Tea

- **Preparation Time:** 5 minutes
- **Serves:** 1

Ingredients:

- 1 chamomile tea bag or 1 tablespoon dried chamomile flowers
- 1 cup hot water
- Honey or lemon (optional, for flavor)

Nutritional Information: Calories: 0 | Carbohydrates: 0g | Caffeine: None

Instructions:

1. Place the chamomile tea bag or dried chamomile flowers in a teacup or mug.

2. Heat water in a kettle or microwave until it reaches boiling point.

3. Pour the hot water over the chamomile tea bag or flowers in the cup.

4. Steep the chamomile tea for about 5 minutes to allow the flavors to infuse.

5. Remove the tea bag or strain out the chamomile flowers.

6. Add honey or a squeeze of lemon if desired for added flavor.

7. Stir well and enjoy the soothing and relaxing Chamomile Tea.

Serving Suggestions:

- Enjoy with a dash of honey or a slice of lemon for added flavor.

Nutrient-Packed Green Smoothie

- **Preparation Time:** 5 minutes
- **Serves:** 1

Ingredients:

- 1 cup unsweetened almond milk or coconut milk
- 1 cup baby spinach or kale leaves
- 1/2 avocado
- 1/2 cup frozen cauliflower florets
- 1 tablespoon chia seeds or ground flaxseeds
- 1/2 teaspoon ground cinnamon

- 1/4 teaspoon vanilla extract
- Stevia or monk fruit sweetener (optional, to taste)

Nutritional Information: Calories: 280, Carbs: 18g, Fiber: 10g, Protein: 8g, Fat: 20g

Instructions:

1. Put all your ingredients into a high-powered blender.

2. Blend on high speed until smooth and creamy.

3. If the smoothie is too thick, add a splash of unsweetened almond or coconut milk to reach the desired consistency.

4. Taste and adjust sweetness with stevia or monk fruit sweetener if desired.

5. Pour into a glass and enjoy immediately.

Serving Suggestions:

- For a pop of color and a burst of citrusy freshness, garnish with a wedge of lemon or lime.

CHAPTER 3

30 Days Meal Plan For Gastroparesis Diet

Please note that the provided meal plan is a sample and should not be interpreted as a recommendation to consume all the listed recipes in a single day.

This meal plan aims to offer inspiration and guidance for healthy meal preparation. Feel free to customize this plan to suit your preferences and dietary requirements.

Day 1:

- **Breakfast:** Vanilla Chia Pudding
- **Lunch:** Miso Soup with Silken Tofu and Seaweed
- **Dinner:** Turkey Meatballs with Pureed Vegetables and Mashed Cauliflower
- **Dessert/Snack:** Avocado Chocolate Mousse
- **Beverage/Drink:** Lemon Ginger Elixir

Day 2:

- **Breakfast:** Warm Rice Cereal with Cinnamon
- **Lunch:** Chicken Lettuce Wraps with Low-Sodium Soy Sauce
- **Dinner:** Baked Tilapia Caesar Salad with Low-Fat Dressing
- **Dessert/Snack:** Homemade Applesauce
- **Beverage/Drink:** Pomegranate Juice

Day 3:

- **Breakfast:** Jicama Toast
- **Lunch:** Zucchini Noodles with Pesto
- **Dinner:** Lentil Soup with Low-Fat Vegetable Broth
- **Dessert/Snack:** Mango Sorbet
- **Beverage/Drink:** Unsweetened Golden Milk

Day 4:

- **Breakfast:** Scrambled Eggs with Spinach and Feta
- **Lunch:** Tuna Salad on Endive Spears
- **Dinner:** Grilled Lean Beef Tenderloin with Garlic Spinach Purée

- **Dessert/Snack:** Lemon Coconut Energy Bites
- **Beverage/Drink:** Chamomile Tea

Day 5:

- **Breakfast:** Papaya "Boats" with Chia Pudding
- **Lunch:** Poached Salmon with Roasted Asparagus and Lemon
- **Dinner:** Beef Stew with Pureed Vegetables and Cauliflower Breadsticks
- **Dessert/Snack:** Pumpkin Custard
- **Beverage/Drink:** Nutrient-Packed Green Smoothie

Day 6:

- **Breakfast:** Melon and Cottage Cheese Medley
- **Lunch:** Pureed Broccoli and Cheddar Soup with Low-Fat Crackers
- **Dinner:** Baked Cod with Lemon Butter Sauce and Quinoa
- **Dessert/Snack:** Avocado Chocolate Mousse
- **Beverage/Drink:** Lemon Ginger Elixir

Day 7:

- **Breakfast:** Poached Pears with Vanilla Bean Ricotta
- **Lunch:** Shrimp Skewers with Roasted Bell Peppers and Couscous
- **Dinner:** Steamed Fish Fillet with Grilled Portobello Mushroom Caps
- **Dessert/Snack:** Homemade Applesauce
- **Beverage/Drink:** Pomegranate Juice

Day 8:

- **Breakfast:** Vanilla Chia Pudding
- **Lunch:** Miso Soup with Silken Tofu and Seaweed
- **Dinner:** Turkey Meatballs with Pureed Vegetables and Mashed Cauliflower
- **Dessert/Snack:** Mango Sorbet
- **Beverage/Drink:** Unsweetened Golden Milk

Day 9:

- **Breakfast:** Warm Rice Cereal with Cinnamon
- **Lunch:** Chicken Lettuce Wraps with Low-Sodium Soy Sauce
- **Dinner:** Baked Tilapia Caesar Salad with Low-Fat Dressing
- **Dessert/Snack:** Lemon Coconut Energy Bites
- **Beverage/Drink:** Chamomile Tea

Day 10:

- **Breakfast:** Jicama Toast
- **Lunch:** Zucchini Noodles with Pesto
- **Dinner:** Lentil Soup with Low-Fat Vegetable Broth
- **Dessert/Snack:** Pumpkin Custard
- **Beverage/Drink:** Nutrient-Packed Green Smoothie

Day 11:

- **Breakfast:** Scrambled Eggs with Spinach and Feta
- **Lunch:** Tuna Salad on Endive Spears
- **Dinner:** Grilled Lean Beef Tenderloin with Garlic Spinach Purée
- **Dessert/Snack:** Avocado Chocolate Mousse

- **Beverage/Drink:** Lemon Ginger Elixir

Day 12:

- **Breakfast:** Papaya "Boats" with Chia Pudding
- **Lunch:** Poached Salmon with Roasted Asparagus and Lemon
- **Dinner:** Beef Stew with Pureed Vegetables and Cauliflower Breadsticks
- **Dessert/Snack:** Homemade Applesauce
- **Beverage/Drink:** Pomegranate Juice

Day 13:

- **Breakfast:** Melon and Cottage Cheese Medley
- **Lunch:** Pureed Broccoli and Cheddar Soup with Low-Fat Crackers
- **Dinner:** Baked Cod with Lemon Butter Sauce and Quinoa
- **Dessert/Snack:** Mango Sorbet
- **Beverage/Drink:** Unsweetened Golden Milk

Day 14:

- **Breakfast:** Poached Pears with Vanilla Bean Ricotta

- **Lunch:** Shrimp Skewers with Roasted Bell Peppers and Couscous
- **Dinner:** Steamed Fish Fillet with Grilled Portobello Mushroom Caps
- **Dessert/Snack:** Lemon Coconut Energy Bites
- **Beverage/Drink:** Chamomile Tea

Day 15:

- **Breakfast:** Vanilla Chia Pudding
- **Lunch:** Miso Soup with Silken Tofu and Seaweed
- **Dinner:** Turkey Meatballs with Pureed Vegetables and Mashed Cauliflower
- **Dessert/Snack:** Pumpkin Custard
- **Beverage/Drink:** Nutrient-Packed Green Smoothie

Day 16:

- **Breakfast:** Warm Rice Cereal with Cinnamon
- **Lunch:** Chicken Lettuce Wraps with Low-Sodium Soy Sauce
- **Dinner:** Baked Tilapia Caesar Salad with Low-Fat Dressing
- **Dessert/Snack:** Avocado Chocolate Mousse
- **Beverage/Drink:** Lemon Ginger Elixir

Day 17:

- **Breakfast:** Jicama Toast
- **Lunch:** Zucchini Noodles with Pesto
- **Dinner:** Lentil Soup with Low-Fat Vegetable Broth
- **Dessert/Snack:** Mango Sorbet
- **Beverage/Drink:** Pomegranate Juice

Day 18:

- **Breakfast:** Scrambled Eggs with Spinach and Feta
- **Lunch:** Tuna Salad on Endive Spears
- **Dinner:** Grilled Lean Beef Tenderloin with Garlic Spinach Purée
- **Dessert/Snack:** Lemon Coconut Energy Bites
- **Beverage/Drink:** Chamomile Tea

Day 19:

- **Breakfast:** Papaya "Boats" with Chia Pudding
- **Lunch:** Poached Salmon with Roasted Asparagus and Lemon
- **Dinner:** Beef Stew with Pureed Vegetables and Cauliflower Breadsticks
- **Dessert/Snack:** Homemade Applesauce
- **Beverage/Drink:** Nutrient-Packed Green Smoothie

Day 20:

- **Breakfast:** Melon and Cottage Cheese Medley
- **Lunch:** Pureed Broccoli and Cheddar Soup with Low-Fat Crackers
- **Dinner:** Baked Cod with Lemon Butter Sauce and Quinoa
- **Dessert/Snack:** Pumpkin Custard
- **Beverage/Drink:** Lemon Ginger Elixir

Day 21:

- **Breakfast:** Poached Pears with Vanilla Bean Ricotta
- **Lunch:** Shrimp Skewers with Roasted Bell Peppers and Couscous
- **Dinner:** Steamed Fish Fillet with Grilled Portobello Mushroom Caps
- **Dessert/Snack:** Avocado Chocolate Mousse
- **Beverage/Drink:** Pomegranate Juice

Day 22:

- **Breakfast:** Vanilla Chia Pudding
- **Lunch:** Miso Soup with Silken Tofu and Seaweed

- **Dinner:** Turkey Meatballs with Pureed Vegetables and Mashed Cauliflower
- **Dessert/Snack:** Lemon Coconut Energy Bites
- **Beverage/Drink:** Chamomile Tea

Day 23:

- **Breakfast:** Warm Rice Cereal with Cinnamon
- **Lunch:** Chicken Lettuce Wraps with Low-Sodium Soy Sauce
- **Dinner:** Baked Tilapia Caesar Salad with Low-Fat Dressing
- **Dessert/Snack:** Homemade Applesauce
- **Beverage/Drink:** Nutrient-Packed Green Smoothie

Day 24:

- **Breakfast:** Jicama Toast
- **Lunch:** Zucchini Noodles with Pesto
- **Dinner:** Lentil Soup with Low-Fat Vegetable Broth
- **Dessert/Snack:** Mango Sorbet
- **Beverage/Drink:** Pomegranate Juice

Day 25:

- **Breakfast:** Scrambled Eggs with Spinach and Feta
- **Lunch:** Tuna Salad on Endive Spears

- **Dinner:** Grilled Lean Beef Tenderloin with Garlic Spinach Purée
- **Dessert/Snack:** Lemon Coconut Energy Bites
- **Beverage/Drink:** Chamomile Tea

Day 26:

- **Breakfast:** Papaya "Boats" with Chia Pudding
- **Lunch:** Poached Salmon with Roasted Asparagus and Lemon
- **Dinner:** Beef Stew with Pureed Vegetables and Cauliflower Breadsticks
- **Dessert/Snack:** Homemade Applesauce
- **Beverage/Drink:** Nutrient-Packed Green Smoothie

Day 27:

- **Breakfast:** Melon and Cottage Cheese Medley
- **Lunch:** Pureed Broccoli and Cheddar Soup with Low-Fat Crackers
- **Dinner:** Baked Cod with Lemon Butter Sauce and Quinoa
- **Dessert/Snack:** Pumpkin Custard
- **Beverage/Drink:** Lemon Ginger Elixir

Day 28:

- **Breakfast:** Poached Pears with Vanilla Bean Ricotta
- **Lunch:** Shrimp Skewers with Roasted Bell Peppers and Couscous
- **Dinner:** Steamed Fish Fillet with Grilled Portobello Mushroom Caps
- **Dessert/Snack:** Avocado Chocolate Mousse
- **Beverage/Drink:** Pomegranate Juice

Day 29:

- **Breakfast:** Vanilla Chia Pudding
- **Lunch:** Miso Soup with Silken Tofu and Seaweed
- **Dinner:** Turkey Meatballs with Pureed Vegetables and Mashed Cauliflower
- **Dessert/Snack:** Mango Sorbet
- **Beverage/Drink:** Unsweetened Golden Milk

Day 30:

- **Breakfast:** Warm Rice Cereal with Cinnamon
- **Lunch:** Chicken Lettuce Wraps with Low-Sodium Soy Sauce
- **Dinner:** Baked Tilapia Caesar Salad with Low-Fat Dressing
- **Dessert/Snack:** Pumpkin Custard
- **Beverage/Drink:** Nutrient-Packed Green Smoothie

CHAPTER 4

Conclusion

You made it! Congratulations on reaching the end of this life-changing culinary journey tailored specifically for those navigating gastroparesis and diabetes.

This book has been your trusted companion, guiding you through the principles and strategies to reclaim the sheer enjoyment of eating without sacrificing your well-being.

Along the way, you've discovered a delicious array of recipes that prove you don't have to compromise flavor for health. Each dish has been thoughtfully crafted to provide maximum nourishment while being gentle on your digestive system and kind to your blood sugar levels.

But this isn't just a cookbook – it's a testament to your resilience and determination to live life to the fullest, savoring every bite without letting gastroparesis or diabetes dictate your dining experience. You've learned that with the right knowledge and mindset, you can transform challenges into opportunities for growth and empowerment.

As you close this book, carry with you the confidence that you now possess the tools to continue this journey with ease.

The recipes you've discovered are merely the beginning – a foundation upon which you can build your own culinary masterpieces, tailored to your unique palate and dietary needs.

Embrace the freedom that comes with understanding your body's requirements, and never hesitate to experiment, adapt, and create new culinary adventures that celebrate your individuality while honoring your well-being.

Remember, every meal is an opportunity to nourish your body, soul, and spirit. Approach each one with a sense of joy and gratitude, for you now have the power to turn every bite into a celebration of life, health, and happiness.

Made in the USA
Columbia, SC
03 July 2024

38038101R20057